REFLECTIONS
ON
CHANGING

GW00363073

Attic Press
Dublin

First published in 1992 by
Attic Press
4 Upper Mount Street
Dublin 2

British Library Cataloguing in Publication Data
A catalogue record for this book is available from the
British Library.

ISBN 1-85594-048-5

Cover Design: Kate White
Origination: Sinéad Bevan, Attic Press
Selection Co-ordinator: Maeve Kneafsey
Printing: Colour Books Ltd, Dublin

Attic Reflections Series

During the past few years we have seen an explosion of interest in the area generally referred to as 'New Age'. This can be seen in the enormous growth in the number of people taking an alternative approach to all aspects of living in the modern world.

The search for new alternatives reaches into the area of spirituality and personal development, with many seeking answers to questions of personal growth outside the more traditional methods.

In response to this need Attic Press is delighted to launch the **ATTIC REFLECTIONS SERIES**.

We will continue to add to this series with relevant and resourceful Reflections.

Beautifully presented and illustrated, these books will be ones you find yourself returning to again and again.

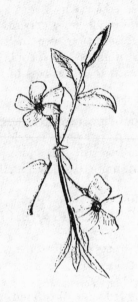

Nobody told me how hard and lonely change is.

Joan Gilbertson

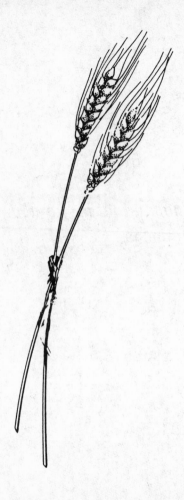

When you put your hand to the plough, you can't put it down until you get to the end of the row.

Alice Paul

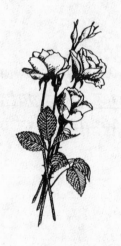

*Change cannot be avoided ... Change
provides the opportunity for
innovation. It gives you the chance
to demonstrate your creativity.*

Felice Jones

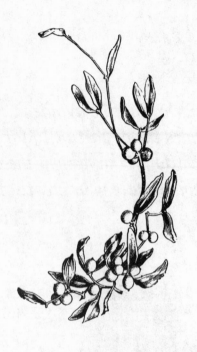

*If you want a place in the sun
you've got to put up with a few
blisters.*

Abigail Van Buren

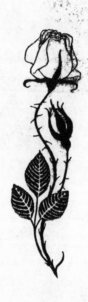

Every thought you have makes up some segment of the world you see. It is with your thoughts, then, that we must work, if your perception of the world is to be changed.

Joanne Smythe

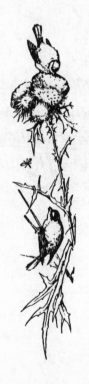

With courage you will dare to take risks, have the strength to be compassionate and the wisdom to be humble. Courage is the foundation of integrity.

Chinese Proverb

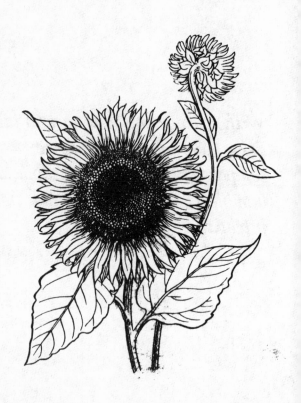

When one door closes another opens. Expect that new door to reveal even greater wonders and glories and surprises. Feel yourself grow with every experience. And look for the reason for it.

Eileen Caddy

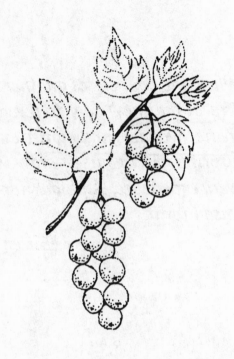

Everyday life confronts us with new problems to be solved, which force us to adjust our old programmes accordingly.

Ann Faraday

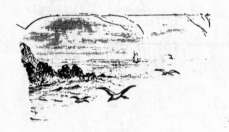

The miracle is not to fly in the air, or to walk on the water, but to walk on the earth.

Chinese Proverb

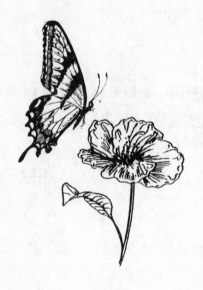

Those interested in perpetuating present conditions are always in tears about the marvellous past that is about to disappear, without having so much as a smile for the young future.

Simone de Beauvoir

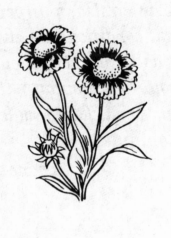

You may believe that you are responsible for what you do, but not for what you think. The truth is that you are responsible for what you think, because it is only at this level that you can exercise choice. What you do comes from what you think.

Joan Greer

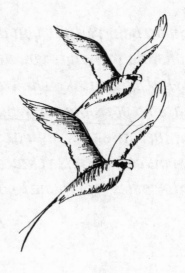

At fifteen, life had taught me undeniably, that surrender, in its place, was as honourable as resistance, especially if one had no choice.

Maya Angelou

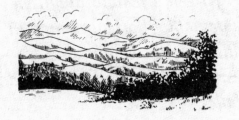

Life is what it is, you cannot change it, but you can change yourself.

French Proverb

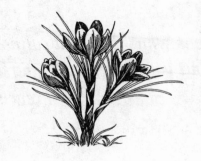

A clay pot sitting in the sun will always be a clay pot. It has to go through the white heat of the furnace to become porcelain.

Mildred Wite Stouven

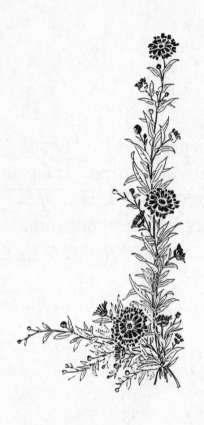

When you get into a tight place and everything goes against you 'till it seems as though you could not hold on a minute longer, never give up then, for that is just the place and time that the tide will turn.

Harriet Beecher Stowe

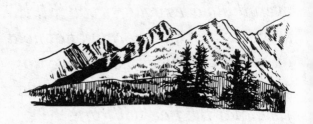

You cannot stay on the summit forever; you have to come down again ... So why bother in the first place? Just this: what is above knows what is below, but what is below does not know what is above.

Reneé Daumal

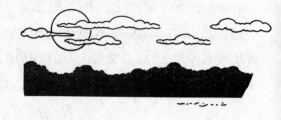

Never measure the height of a mountain, until you have reached the top. Then you will see how low it was.

Danish Proverb

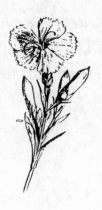

All we are asked to bear we can bear. That is a law of the spiritual life. The only hindrance to the work of this law, as of all benign laws, is fear.

Elizabeth Goudge

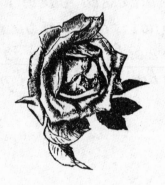

Everything is so dangerous that nothing is really very frightening.

Gertrude Stein

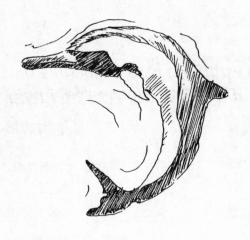

*Have no fear
of moving into the unknown.
Simply step out fearlessly
knowing that I am with you,
therefore no harm can befall you;
all is very well.
Do this in complete faith
and confidence.*

Eileen Caddy

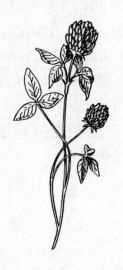

Life is a series
of natural
and spontaneous
changes.
Don't resist them -
that only creates sorrow.
Let reality be reality.
Let things flow naturally forward
in whatever way
they will.

Lao-Tse

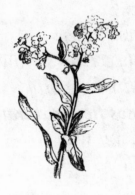

The secret of making
something work in your life is,
first of all,
the deep desire to make it work:
than the faith and belief
that it can work:
then to hold that clear definite
vision in your consciousness
and see it working out
step by step,
without one thought
of doubt or disbelief.

Eileen Caddy

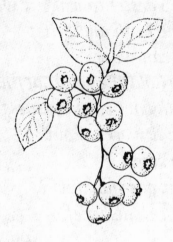

I have a clear choice between life and death, between reality and fantasy, between health and sickness.
I have to become responsible - responsible for mistakes as well as accomplishments.

Eileen Mayhew

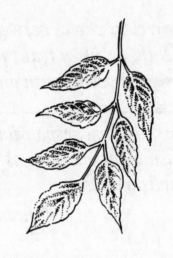

You are given the gifts of the gods;
you create your reality
according to your beliefs.
Yours is the creative energy
that makes your world.
There are no limitations
to the self
except those you believe in.

                                    Jane Roberts

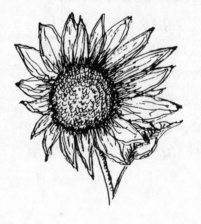

*Life is either
a daring adventure
or nothing.*

Helen Keller

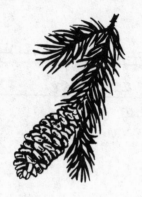

Trials are but lessons
that you failed to learn
presented once again,
so where you made a faulty choice
before, you can now make a better
one and thus escape all pain
that what you chose before
has brought to you.

Russian Proverb

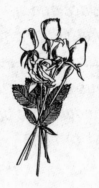

There are
always risks
in freedom.
The only risk
in bondage
is that
of breaking free.

Gita Bellin

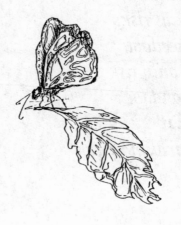

Stop sitting there
with your hands folded
looking on, doing nothing;
Get into action
and live this full
and glorious life.
Now.
You have to do it.

Eileen Caddy

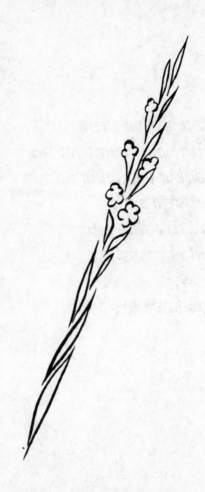

Life is like a wild tiger.
You can either lie down
and let it
Lay its paw on your head -
Or sit on its back and ride it.

Indian Proverb

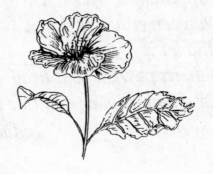

Every time we say
'I must do something'
it takes an incredible
amount of energy.
Far more
than physically
doing it.

Gita Bellin

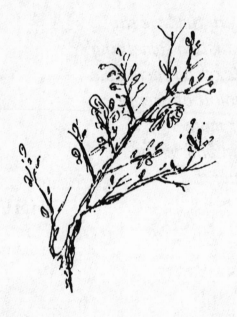

I do not want to die ... until I have
faithfully made the most of my
talent
and cultivated the seed that was
placed in me, until the last small
twig
has grown.

Kathe Kollwitz

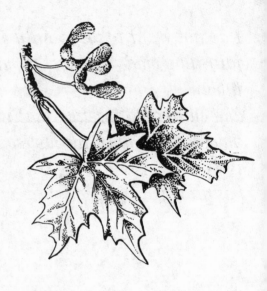

You are never asked
to do more than you are able
without being given
the strength and ability
to do it.

Eileen Caddy

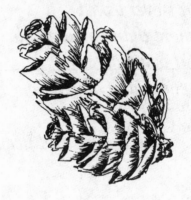

Before enlightenment
chopping wood
carrying water.
After enlightenment
chopping wood
carrying water.

Zen Proverb

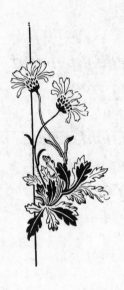

Be like a very small
joyous child
living gloriously in the
ever present now
without a single
worry or concern
about even the next
moment of time.

Eileen Caddy

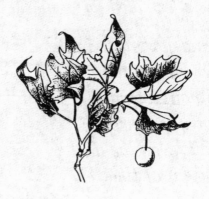

Even though I have my share of
storm with everyone else, I am
comforted always by the knowledge
that there is land below, because I
have seen it. I am inspired to go on
because I have seen the meaning
myself.

Sylvia Ashton-Warner

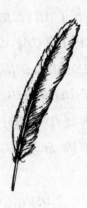

It is not because things are difficult that we do not dare; it is because we do not dare that they are difficult.

Chinese Proverb

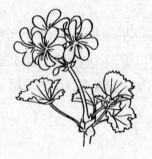

The bottom line is that I am
responsible for my own well being,
my own happiness.
The choices and decisions I make
regarding my life, directly influence
the quality of my days.

Kathleen Andrus

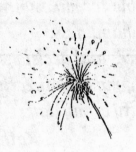

Regrets
can hold you back
and can prevent the most
wonderful things
taking place
in your
life.

Eileen Caddy

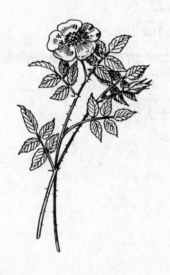

... as the springs return -
regardless of time
so is hope!
Sometimes but a tiny bud
that has to push up
through the hard shell
of circumstance
to reach the light
of accomplishment.
Do not give up HOPE!

                    Dorothy Miller Cole

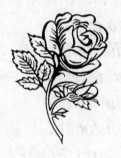

*Stop looking
for a scapegoat
in your life
but be willing
to face the truth
within yourself
and right
your own wrongs.*

Eileen Caddy

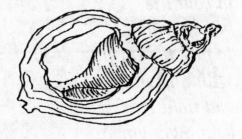

But now all I need in order to have a future, is to design a future I can manage to get inside of.

Francine Julian Clark

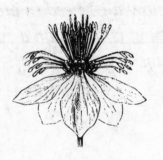

The future belongs to those who believe in the beauty of their dreams.

Eleanor Roosevelt

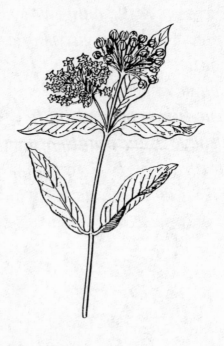

There are really only two ways to
approach life: as victim or as gallant
fighter.
You must decide if you want to act
or react.
Deal your own cards or play with a
stacked deck.
And if you don't decide which way
to play with life, it always plays
with you.

                    Merle Shain

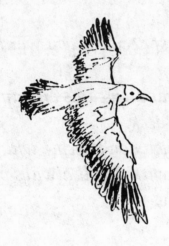

I see life sometimes as a bird flying. I see a soul on the wing through a trackless storm, and every now and again there is a lull and the bird comes to rest on land. These contacts with the earth before departing into the storm again I see as the moments in life when I know the meaning.

Sylvia Ashton-Warner

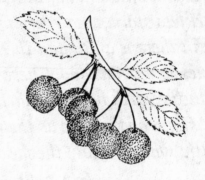

That which has been
done to us
we do to others ...
unless we heal our past.

Jane Smythe

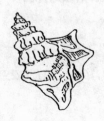

*What you do in life is
vaguely interesting;
Who you are is inspiring.*

Rita Hogarth

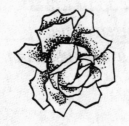

Life is a process of becoming, a combination of states we have to go through. Where people fail is that they wish to elect a state and remain in it. This is a kind of death.

Anais Nin

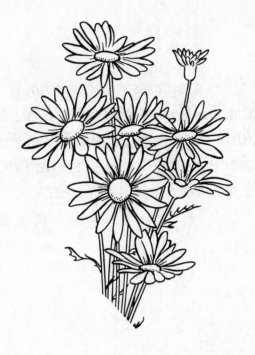

Trust.
But trust that it will all turn
out perfectly, not that others will
necessarily do what you expect
them to do.

Rita Hogarth

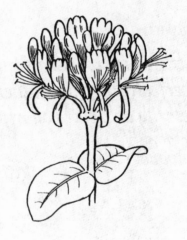

*See every difficulty
as a challenge,
a stepping stone,
and never be defeated
by anything
or anyone.*

Eileen Caddy

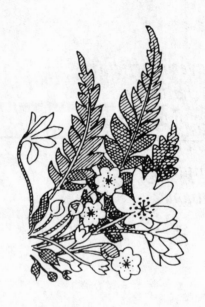

I'm suddenly realising that I've
wasted a lot of time just being afraid
just being polite and just holding
back and just letting people do just
what they want with us.

Mary Tsukamoto

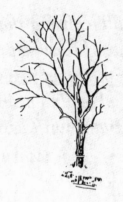

An ox at the roadside, when it is dying of hunger and thirst, does not lie down; it walks up and down - up and down, seeking it knows not what - but it does not lie down.

Olive Schreiner

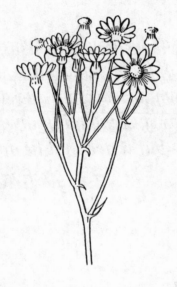

Walls have been built against us, but we are always fighting to tear them down, and in the fighting, we grow, we find new strength, new scope.

Eslanda Gode Robeson

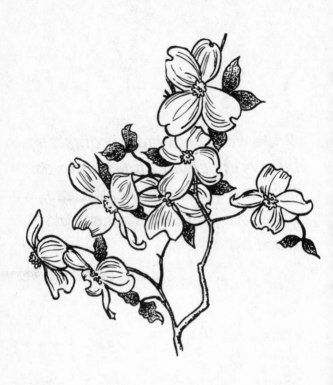

Until we can all present ourselves to the world in our completeness, as fully and beautifully as we see ourselves naked in our bedrooms, we are not free.

Merie Woo

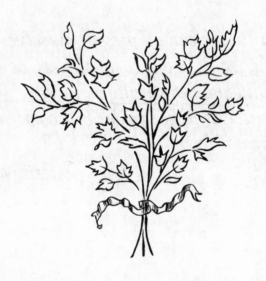

The most frustrating thing about unwelcome and chronic pain is its mandate to revise your life. Revision marks a measure of acceptance. And to accept it feels too much like abandoning independence.

Carolyn Hardesty

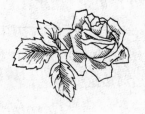

When you feel
that you have reached the end
and that you cannot go
one step further,
when life seems to be
drained of all purpose:
What a wonderful opportunity
to start all over again,
to turn over a new page.

Eileen Caddy

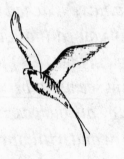

Lifting as they climb, onward and upward they go struggling and striving and hoping that the buds and blossoms of their desires may burst into glorious fruition ere long.

Mary Church Terrell

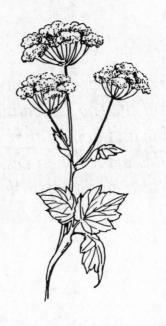

Apparent failure may hold in its rough shell the germs of a success that will blossom in time, and bear fruit throughout eternity.

Frances Ellen Harper

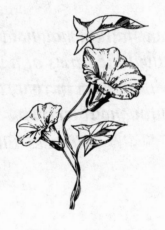

I always wanted to be somebody. If I made it, it's half because I was game enough to take a lot of punishment along the way and half because there were a lot of people who cared enough to help me.

Althea Gibson

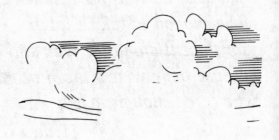

Instead of trying to change situations, have them the way they are.
That is the only way they are going to change.

Rita Hogarth

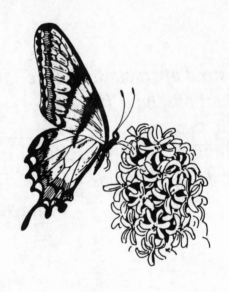

The way it turns out
is the way
you intend it to turn out
even though you
may not want
it that way.

Jane Smythe

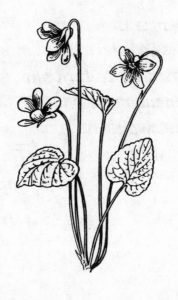

Changes (in life) are not only possible and predictable, but to deny them is to be an accomplice to one's own unnecessary vegetation.

Gail Sheehy

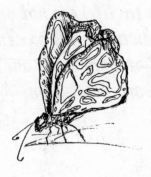

People change and forget to tell each other.

> *Lillian Hellman*

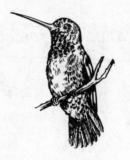

Learning moment by moment to be free in our minds and hearts, we make freedom possible for everyone the world over.

Sonia Johnson

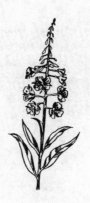

If you have enough fantasies, you're ready, in the event that something happens.

Sheila Ballantyne

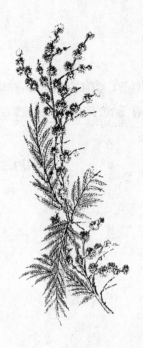

Follow your dream ... take one step at a time and don't settle for less, just continue to climb.

Amanda Bradley

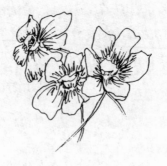

Dwell not on the past.
Use it to illustrate a point,
then leave it behind.
Nothing really matters
except what you do now
in this instant of time.
From this moment onward
you can be an entirely different
person, filled with love and
understanding,
ready with an outstretched hand,
uplifted and positive
in every thought
and deed.

Eileen Caddy

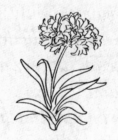

When a woman tells the truth she is creating the possibility for more truth around her.

Adrienne Rich

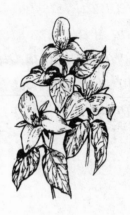

When I am all hassled about something, I always stop and ask myself what difference it will make in the evolution of the human species in the next ten million years, and that question always helps me to get back my perspective.

Anne Wilson Schaef

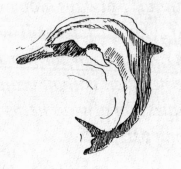

It is important
from time to time
to slow down,
to go away by yourself,
and simply
Be.

Eileen Caddy

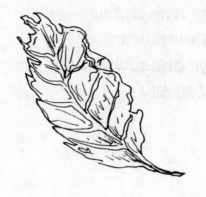

It is very easy to forgive others their mistakes. It takes more gut and gumption to forgive them for having witnessed your own.

Jessamyn West

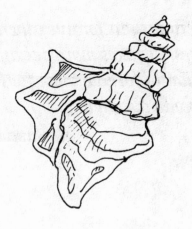

Living in process is being open to insight and encounter. Creativity is becoming intensively absorbed in the process and giving it form.

Susan Smith

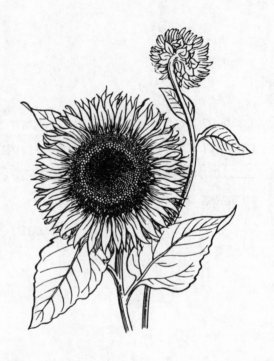

Make it a rule of life never to regret and never look back. Regret is an appalling waste of energy; you can't build on it; it is good only for wallowing in.

Katherine Mansfield

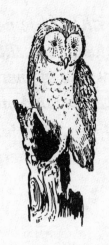

We are not human beings trying to be spiritual. We are spiritual beings trying to be human.

Jacquelyn Small

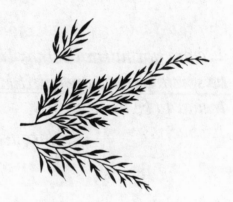

Our most important decisions are discovered, not made. We can make the unimportant ones but the major ones require us to wait with the discovery.

Anne Wilson Schaef

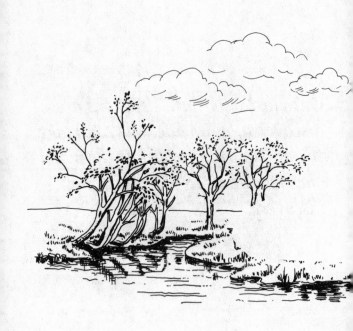

The clouds gathered together, stood still and watched the river scuttle around the forest floor, crash headlong into haunches of hills with no notion of where it was going, until exhausted, ill and grieving, it slowed to a stop just twenty leagues short of the sea.

Toni Morrison

Long term change requires looking honestly at our lives and realising that it's nice to be needed, but not at the expense of our health, our happiness, and our sanity.

Ellen Sue Stern

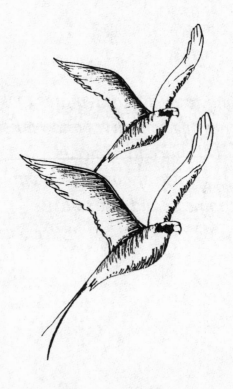

The way forward is to acknowledge our partnership with everyone.

Rita Hogarth

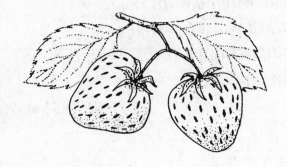

Yesterday is a cancelled cheque
Tomorrow is a promissory note
Today is cash in hand, spend it
wisely.

May Updike

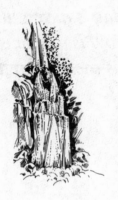

As long as we think dug-out canoes
are the only possibility - we will
never see the ship, we will never feel
the wind blow.

Sonia Johnson

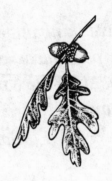

Life was meant to be lived and curiosity must be kept alive. One must never, for whatever reason, turn one's back on life.

Eleanor Roosevelt

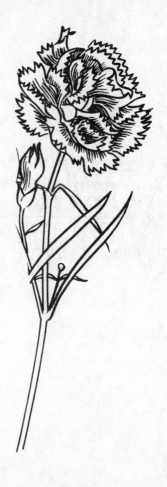

The events in our lives happen in a sequence in time, but in their significance to ourselves, they find their own order ... the continuous thread of revelation.

Eudora Welty

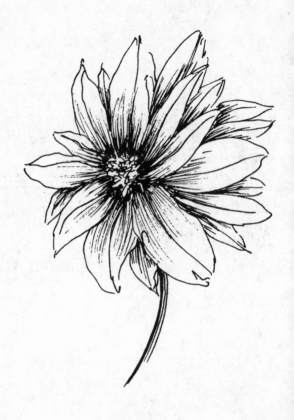

Do nothing because it is righteous or praiseworthy or noble to do so; do nothing because it seems good to do so; do only that which you must do and which you cannot do in any other way.

Ursula K Le Guin

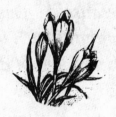

*One needs something to believe in,
something for which one can have
whole-hearted enthusiasm. One
needs to feel that one's life has
meaning, that one is needed in this
world.*

Hannah Senesh

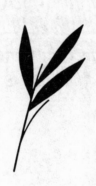

Can I learn to control resentment
and hostility, the ambivalence, born
somewhere far below the conscious
level? If I cannot, I shall lose the
person I love.

May Sarton

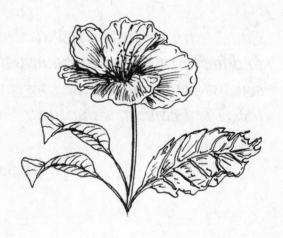

I'm not going to limit myself just because people won't accept the fact that I can do something else.

Dolly Parton

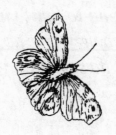

We flood our minds with words! They mesmerise and manipulate us, masking the truth, even when it's set down squarely in front of us. To discover the underlying reality, I've learned to listen only to the action.

Judith M Knowlton

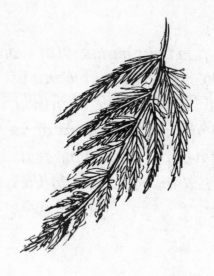

As awareness increases, the need for personal secrecy almost proportionately decreases.

Charlotte Painter

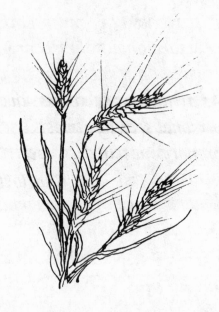

Discoveries have reverberations. A new idea about oneself or some aspect of one's relations to others unsettles all one's other ideas, even the superficially related ones. No matter how slightly, it shifts one's entire orientation. And somewhere along the line of consequences, it changes one's behaviour.

Patricia McLaughlin

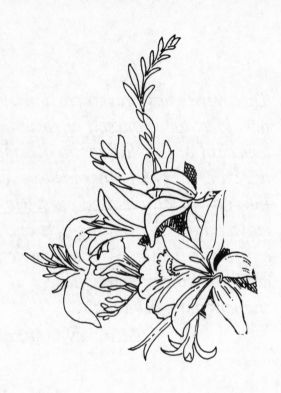

The two important things I did learn
were that you are as powerful and
strong as you allow yourself to be,
and that the most difficult part of
any endeavour is taking the first
step, making the first decision.

Robyn Davidson

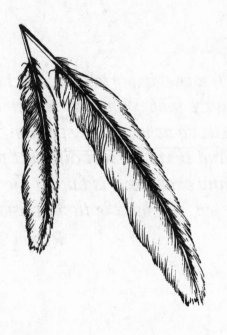

Hope is the thing with feathers
That perches in the soul ...
And sings the tune without words
And ever stops ... at all.

Emily Dickinson

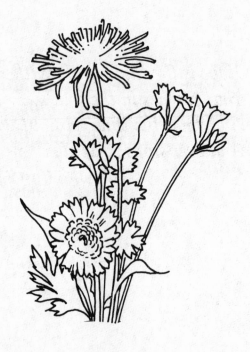

What I am actually saying is that we each need to let our intuition guide us, and then be willing to follow that guidance directly and fearlessly.

Taos Gawain

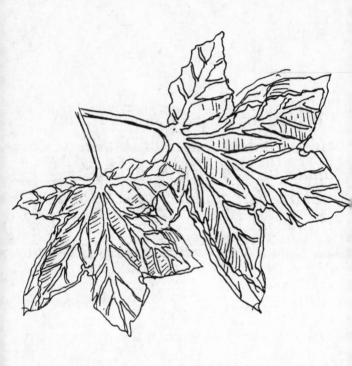

Learn to get in touch with silence within yourself and know that everything in this life has a purpose. There are no mistakes, no coincidences, all events are blessings given to us to learn from.

Elizabeth Kübler-Ross

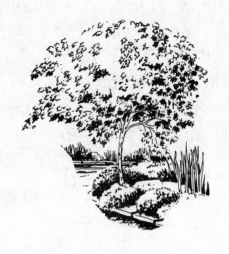

You have to ask the questions and attempt to find answers, because you're right in the middle of it; they've put you in charge - and during a hurricane, too.

Sheila Ballantyne

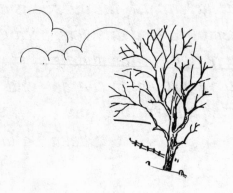

To appreciate openness, we must have experienced encouragement to try the new, to seek alternatives, to view fresh possibilities.

Sister Mary Luke Tobin

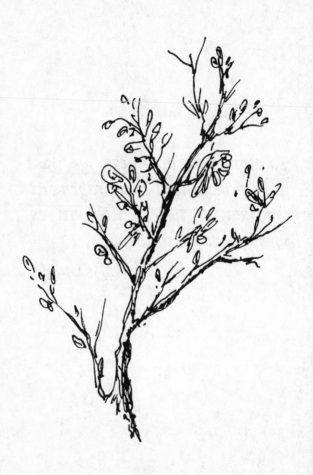

Each of us wants to be significant to someone else. As we are - we're significant to all the lives we're touching at this very moment.

Karen Casey

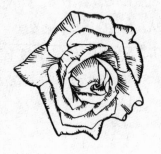

Take your life in your own hands,
and what happens?
A terrible thing; no one to blame.

Erica Jong

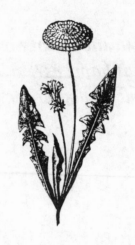

There are two entirely opposite
attitudes possible in facing the
problems of one's life.
One, to try and change the
external world.
The other, to try and change oneself.

Joanna Field

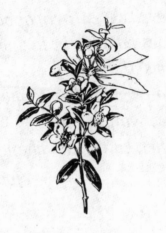

All choices involve risk.
All arouse fear.
Sometimes, when the fear is
experienced as intolerable,
new babies are conceived,
thus postponing the need for change.
Sheila Ballantyne

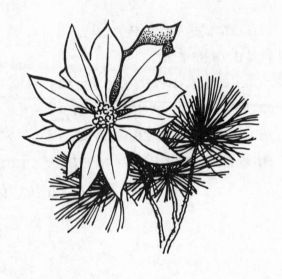

When I am alone the flowers are really seen; I can pay attention to them. They are felt presences. Without them I would die. Why do I say that? Partly because they change before my eyes. They live and die in a few days; they keep me closely in touch with the process, with growth, and also with dying. I am floated on their moments.

May Sarton

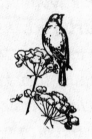

Confidence, that popinjay,
Is planning now
to slip away.
Look fast
it's fading rapidly.
Tomorrow it returns to me.

Maya Angelou

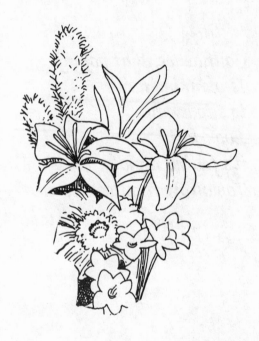

When I keep putting something off, it may not be procrastination, but a decision I've already made and not yet admitted to myself.

Judith M Knowlton

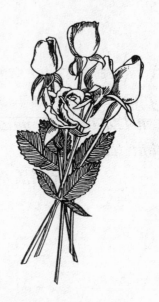

Believing in our hearts that who we are is enough is the key to a more satisfying and balanced life.

Ellen Sue Stern

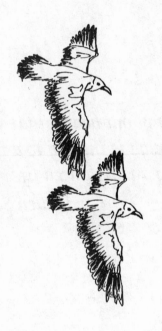

We will discover the nature of our particular genius when we stop trying to conform to our own or to other people's models, learn to be ourselves, and allow our natural channel to open.

Taos Gawain

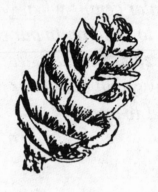

All things are possible until they are proved impossible - and even the impossible may only be so as of now.

Pearl S Buck

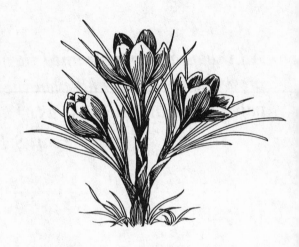

Although the world is very full of suffering, it is also full of the overcoming of it.

Helen Keller

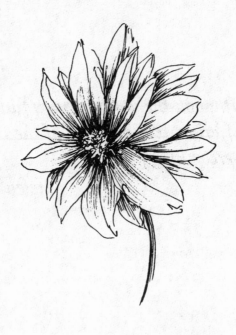

Life is easier to take than you'd think: all that is necessary is to accept the impossible, do without the indispensable and bear the intolerable.

Kathleen Norris

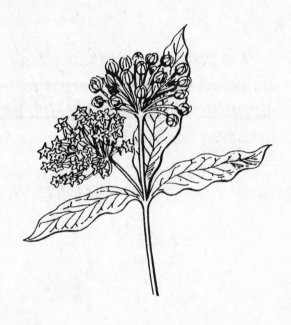

I used to believe that anything was better than nothing. Now I know that sometimes nothing is better.

Glenda Jackson

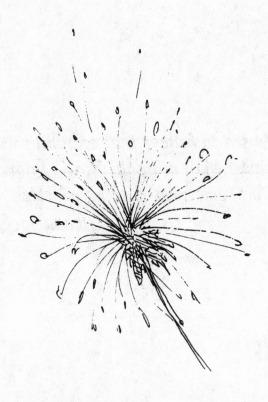

What is the use of such terrible diligence as many tire themselves out with, if they always postpone their exchange of smiles with Beauty and Joy to cling to irksome duties and relations?

Helen Keller

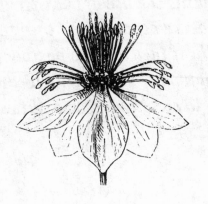

Faults shared are comfortable as bedroom slippers and as easy to slip into.

Phyllis McGinly

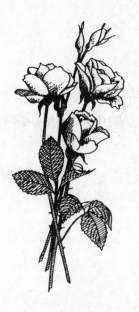

Self-restraint may be alien to the human temperament, but humanity without restraint will dig its own grave.

Myra Mannes

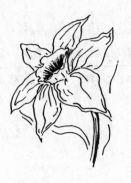

Laughter is much more important than applause. Applause is almost a duty. Laughter is a reward.

Carol Channing

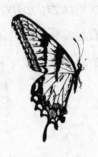

Intimacy with another is a necessary risk if we're to know love. This means loving enough to let someone in on our most hidden parts, daring to share the awful truths about ourselves.

Karen Casey

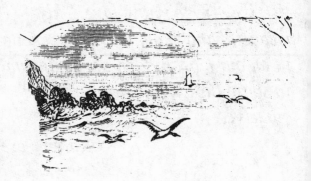

Shall I take you with me?
Shall we go together
All the way to silence,
All the way to land's end?
Is there a choice?

                              May Sarton

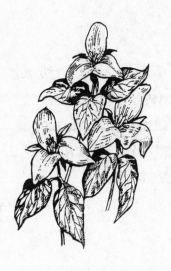

Fickle comfort steals away
what it knows
it will not say
what it can
it will do
it flies from me
to humour you

Maya Angelou

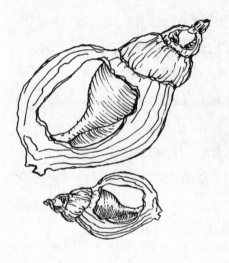

Be at peace
and see
a clear pattern and plan
running through
all your lives.
Nothing is by chance.

Eileen Caddy

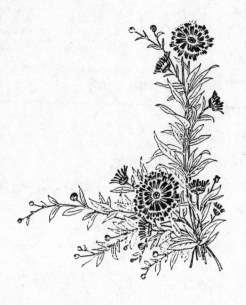

Like an old gold-panning prospector, you must resign yourself to digging up a lot of sand from which you will later patiently wash out a few minute particles of gold ore.

> Dorothy Bryant

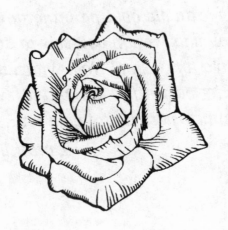

Instead of concentrating on why we can't do a thing, we would be wise to change our 'yes, but ...' attitude to a more positive one. Saying 'yes' means I really do want to change my life for the better.

Liane Cordes

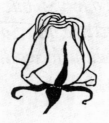

There are as many ways to live and grow as there are people. Our own ways are the only ways that should matter to us.

Evelyn Mandel

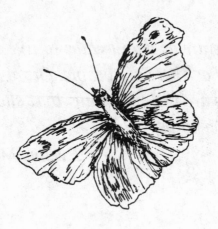

When people make changes in their lives in a certain area, they may start by changing the way they talk about that subject, how they act about it, their attitude toward it, or an underlying decision concerning it.

Jane Clark

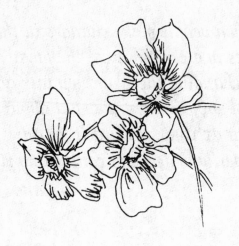

We have seen too much defeatism, too much pessimism, too much of a negative approach. The answer is simple: if you want something very badly, you can achieve it. It may take patience, very hard work, a real struggle, and a long time; but it can be done ... faith is a prerequisite of any undertaking.

Margo Jones

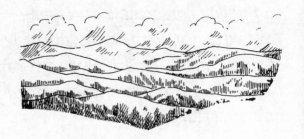

No trumpet sounds when the important decisions of our life are made. Destiny is made known silently.

Agnes de Mille

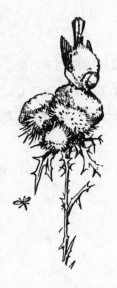

Life is made up of desires that seem big and vital one minute, and little and absurd the next. I guess we get what's best for us in the end.

Alice Caldwell Rice

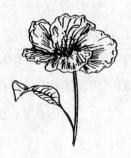

Parents can only give good advice or put one on the right paths, but the final forming of a person's character lies in their own hands.

Anne Frank

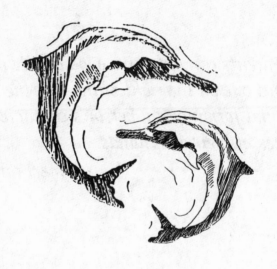

I want to get you excited about who you are, what you are, what you have, and what can still be for you. I want to inspire you to see that you can go far beyond where you are right now.

Virginia Satir

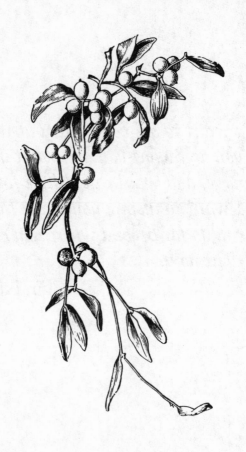

To believe in something not yet proven and to underwrite it with our lives; it is the only way we can leave the future open.

Lillian Smith

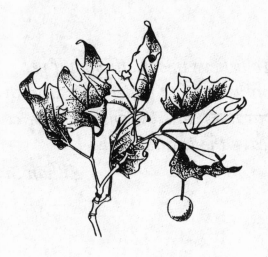

The world is a wheel always
turning. Those who are high go
down low, and those who've been
low go up higher.

Anzia Yezierska

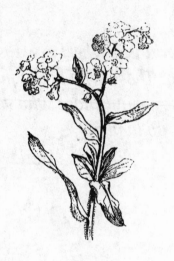

To look backward for a while is to refresh the eye, to restore it, and to render it the more fit for its prime function of looking forward.

Margaret Fairless Barber

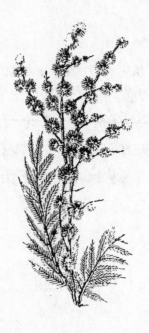

The rare and beautiful experiences of divine revelation are moments of special gifts. Each of us, however, lives each day with special gifts which are a part of our very being, and life is a process of discovering and developing these God-given gifts within each one of us.

Jeane Dixon

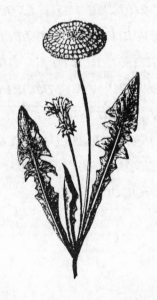

It's ironic, but until you can free those final monsters within the jungle of yourself, your life, your soul is up for grabs.

Rona Barrett

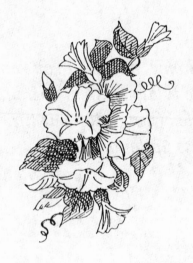

Out of every crisis comes the chance to be reborn, to reconceive ourselves as individuals, to choose the kind of change that will help us to grow and to fulfil ourselves more completely.

Nena O'Neill

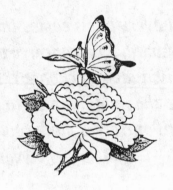

That reality of life and living -
movement from one place to another
either in a project or in a state of
mind, does not conform with what
we imagine or expect or think we
deserve so we often leave things
hanging unfinished or unstarted.

Sandra Edwards

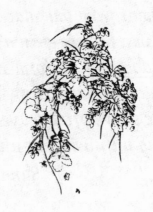

One of the conclusions I have come to in my old age is the importance of living in the ever-present now. In the past, too often I indulged in the belief that somehow or other tomorrow would be brighter or happier or richer.

Ruth Casey

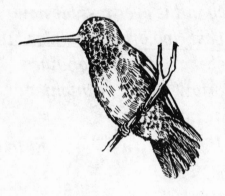

All the fantasies in your life will never match those I once tried to attain. Now older, it's more important reaching the more realistic goals, and having them come true.

Deidra Sarault

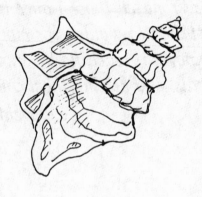

Change occurs when one becomes
what she is, not when she tries to
become what she is not.

Ruth P Freedman

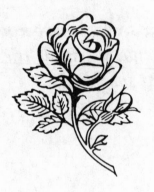

To do nothing is failure. To try, and in the end trying you make some mistakes and then you make some positive changes as a result of those mistakes, is to learn and to grow and to blossom.

Darlene Larson Jenks

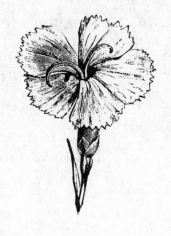

Somewhere along the line of development we discover what we really are, and then we make our real decisions for which we are responsible. Make that decision primarily for yourself because you can never really live anyone else's life, not even your own child's. The influence you exert is through your own life and what you become yourself.

Eleanor Roosevelt

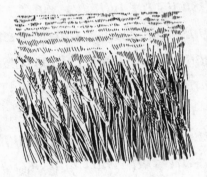

Follow your dream ... if you stumble,
don't stop and lose sight of your
goal, press on to the top.
For only on top
Can we see the whole view ... .

Amanda Bradley

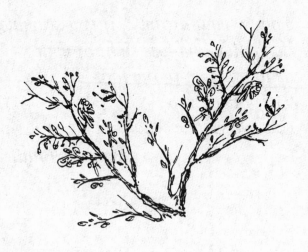

Self-pity in its early stages is as snug as a feather mattress. Only when it hardens does it become uncomfortable.

Maya Angelou

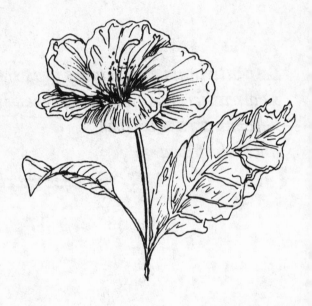

I long to accomplish a great and noble task, but it is my chief duty to accomplish small tasks, as if they were great and noble.

Helen Keller

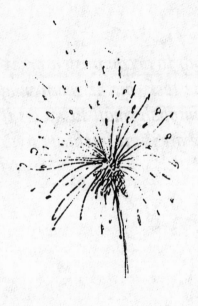

When it comes time to do your own life, you either perpetuate your childhood or you stand on it and finally kick it out from under.

Rosellen Brown

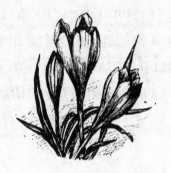

Having spent the better part of my life trying to relive the past or experience the future before it arrives, I have come to believe that in between these two extremes is peace.

Joy Flood

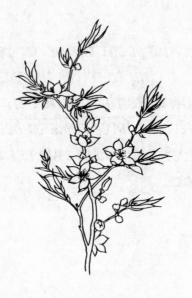

The one important thing I have learned over the years is the difference between taking one's work seriously and taking one's self seriously. The first is imperative and the second is disastrous.

Margot Fonteyn

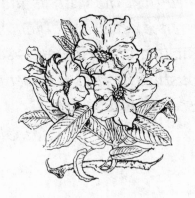

You're wondering if I'm lonely:
OK then, yes, I'm lonely
as a plane rides lonely and level
on its radio beams, aiming
across the Rockies
for the blue-strung aisles
of an airfield on the ocean.

Adrienne Rich

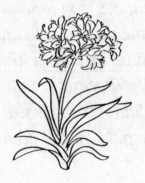

The only sense that is common in the long run, is the sense of change - and we all instinctively avoid it.

E B White

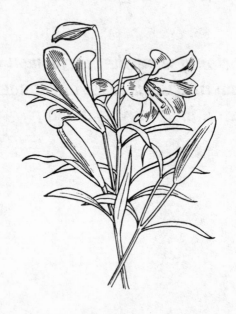

I'm a survivor. Being a survivor doesn't mean you have to be made out of steel and it doesn't mean you have to be ruthless. It means you are basically on your own side and you want to win.

Linda Ronstadt

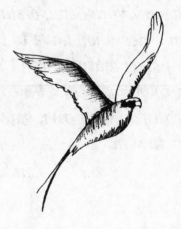

It is good to have an end
to journey towards,
but it is the journey that matters,
in the end.

Ursula K Le Guin

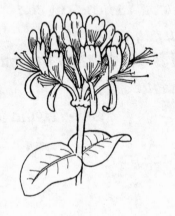

It only takes one person to change your life - you.

Ruth Casey

Keyword Index

300

Author Index